THE MEDICINAL PROPERTIES OF BITTER KOLA AND ITS POTENTIAL HEALTH BENEFITS

THE UNDISCOVERED CAPABILITIES OF BITTER KOLA

EGBO DANIEL

ISBN-13: 9798320248547

Cover design by: Art Painter
Library of Congress Control Number: 2018675309
Printed in the United States of America

This Book is dedicated to God for the ability and enablement to embark and conclude on this piece.

His grace and Love keeps me up and well.

"From Ancient Rituals to Modern Miracles: Unlocking the Wellness Potential of Kolanut"

EGBO DANIEL

CONTENTS

FOREWORD

Within the vast tapestry of nature's gifts lies the bitter kolanut, a symbol of vitality deeply ingrained in West African traditions. In this exploration of its health benefits, we bridge ancient wisdom with modern science, uncovering its potential to nourish both body and spirit.

Through these pages, we delve into its significance in indigenous rituals and its promise as a source of wellness. Yet, beyond its physical attributes, the bitter kolanut reminds us of our interconnectedness with nature and the importance of preserving cultural heritage.

Join us on this journey of discovery, where tradition meets innovation, and the story of the bitter kolanut reveals profound insights into human health and our relationship with the natural world.

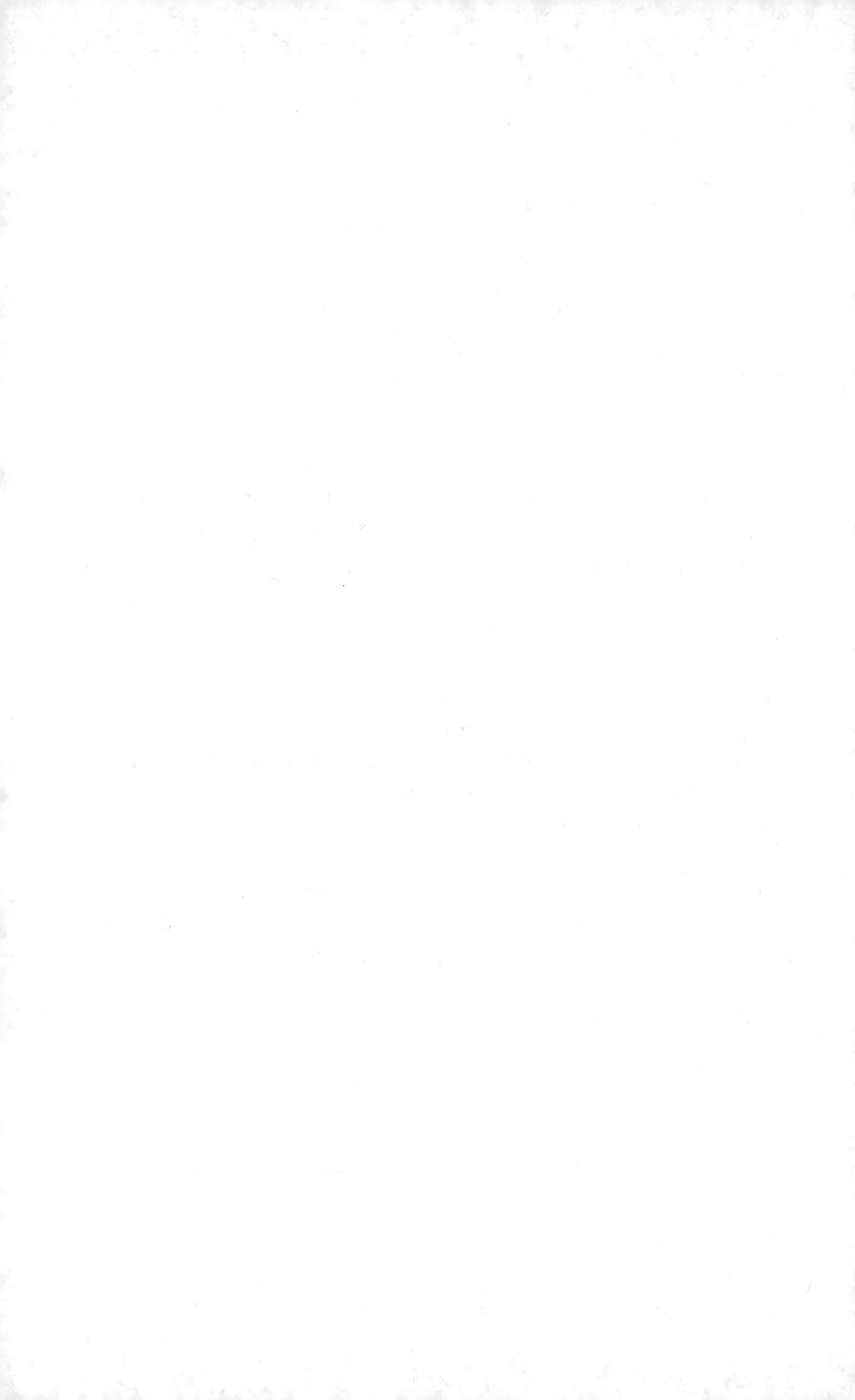

INTRODUCTION

In the heart of the lush rainforests of West and Central Africa, nestled amidst towering trees and teeming biodiversity, lies a remarkable botanical treasure: bitter kola. This humble fruit, scientifically known as Garcinia kola, has been revered for centuries by indigenous communities for its myriad of medicinal properties and cultural significance. From its ancient roots in traditional healing practices to its modern exploration in scientific laboratories, bitter kola continues to captivate the imagination and intrigue researchers, herbalists, and health enthusiasts alike.

The exploration of bitter kola transcends mere botanical curiosity; it delves into the rich tapestry of human history and the enduring relationship between nature and medicine. Throughout the ages, indigenous peoples across Africa have incorporated bitter kola into their healing rituals and herbal remedies, attributing to it an array of curative powers and mystical qualities. Whether used to alleviate ailments, ward off evil spirits, or enhance cognitive function, bitter kola has woven itself into the fabric of cultural traditions, becoming an integral part of the collective consciousness of diverse communities.

Yet, beyond its cultural significance, bitter kola harbors a wealth of biochemical riches waiting to be unlocked. Within its bitter-sweet kernels lie a myriad of phytochemicals, including potent alkaloids, flavonoids, and tannins, each holding the promise of therapeutic potential. Modern scientific inquiry has begun to unravel the intricate pharmacological properties of bitter kola, shedding light on its antioxidant, anti-inflammatory, and antimicrobial effects. As researchers continue to peel back the layers of its botanical mysteries, bitter kola stands poised on the threshold of new discoveries, offering tantalizing glimpses into the realm of natural medicine.

Against the backdrop of a rapidly changing world, where the allure of synthetic drugs often overshadows the wisdom of traditional remedies, the resurgence of interest in bitter kola signals a reawakening of appreciation for nature's pharmacy. As we confront global health challenges, from the rise of antibiotic resistance to the burden of chronic diseases, bitter kola emerges as a beacon of hope—a reminder of the untapped potential lying dormant within the bosom of the natural world.

Through this book, we embark on a journey of discovery—a journey that traverses continents and centuries, weaving together threads of history, culture, science, and tradition. From the ancient rituals of indigenous healers to the cutting-edge research of modern laboratories, we unravel the secrets of bitter kola, exploring its past, present, and future. Join me as we delve into the depths of this botanical marvel, uncovering the stories, science, and spirit of bitter kola—a testament to the enduring power of plants to heal, nourish, and inspire.

Welcome to the world of bitter kola—a journey of exploration, enlightenment, and empowerment.

PREFACE

In this book, we embark on an exploration of the rich and diverse world of kola nut and its profound impact on human health and well-being.

The kola nut, derived from the evergreen kola tree native to the tropical rainforests of West Africa, has a long history of cultural significance and medicinal use. Traditionally revered for its stimulating properties and symbolic value in various cultural practices, the kola nut has also captured the attention of modern science due to its impressive array of health benefits.

As the demand for natural remedies and holistic approaches to wellness continues to grow, the kola nut emerges as a compelling subject of study and fascination. From its role in traditional medicine to its potential applications in modern healthcare, the kola nut offers a wealth of opportunities for exploration and discovery.

In this book, we delve into the scientific research and anecdotal evidence surrounding the health benefits of kola nut. We explore its nutritional profile, phytochemical composition, and physiological effects on the human body. From its antioxidant properties to its potential role in cognitive enhancement and weight management, we uncover the multifaceted ways in which kola nut can contribute to overall health and vitality.

Moreover, we acknowledge the cultural significance of kola nut and its place in various traditions and ceremonies across Africa and beyond. Through the lens of anthropology and cultural studies, we examine the cultural context surrounding the consumption of kola nut and its symbolic importance in social gatherings, rituals, and celebrations.

It is my hope that this book serves as a comprehensive guide to understanding the health benefits of kola nut and inspires further research and exploration into its potential applications in healthcare and wellness. Whether you are a healthcare professional, a researcher, or simply someone curious about the wonders of nature, I invite you to join me on this journey of discovery.

Thank you for embarking on this exploration with me.

EGBO DANIEL

PROLOGUE

In the heart of dense, emerald jungles where sunlight filters through the canopy, and the melody of wildlife fills the air, lies a treasure revered for its potent properties and rich heritage. This treasure, known as the bitter kolanut, transcends its humble appearance to embody a symbol of resilience, cultural significance, and, most importantly, health.

For centuries, indigenous communities of West Africa have held the bitter kolanut in high esteem, recognizing its profound impact on both physical well-being and communal rituals. Passed down through generations, its legacy is woven into the tapestry of local traditions, serving as a cornerstone of vitality and connection.

Yet, beyond its ceremonial role, the bitter kolanut harbors a trove of health benefits waiting to be uncovered by those beyond the jungle's grasp. Concealed within its astringent shell lies a potent fusion of nutrients and bioactive compounds, each holding the promise of enhanced wellness and vitality.

As we embark on this journey of exploration, traversing the realms of scientific inquiry and cultural heritage, let us unveil the secrets of the bitter kolanut—a testament to nature's bounty and the wisdom of generations past. Within its unassuming exterior lies a wealth of potential, offering not only physical nourishment but also a deeper connection to the ancient rhythms of the land.

CAPTER 1: THE HISTORY AND CULTURAL SIGNIFICANCE OF BITTER KOLA

Origins And Distribution

Bitter kola, a botanical marvel native to the tropical rainforests of West and Central Africa, traces its origins back thousands of years. Its natural habitat spans a vast geographical range, encompassing countries such as Nigeria, Cameroon, Ghana, and the Democratic Republic of the Congo. Within these lush and biodiverse ecosystems, bitter kola thrives in the shade of towering trees, its glossy leaves and orange-hued fruits adding splashes of color to the verdant landscape.

Archaeological evidence suggests that bitter kola has been an integral part of African culture since antiquity. Ancient artifacts, such as pottery shards and stone tools, bear witness to its presence in the diet and daily life of indigenous peoples, serving as a source of sustenance, medicine, and spiritual significance. As one of the oldest cultivated plants in the region, bitter kola embodies the enduring relationship between humans and their environment, reflecting a profound understanding of the interconnectedness of all living things.

Cultural Importance And Traditional Uses

In traditional African societies, bitter kola holds a revered place as a symbol of vitality, resilience, and spiritual protection. Its bitter-sweet kernels are imbued with a plethora of symbolic meanings, representing fertility, abundance, and the cyclical rhythms of nature. From birth rituals to marriage ceremonies, bitter kola plays a central role in cultural practices, serving as a tangible expression of communal values and beliefs.

At the heart of bitter kola's cultural significance lies its esteemed reputation as a potent healing agent. For centuries, indigenous healers and herbalists have harnessed its medicinal properties to treat a wide array of ailments, ranging from common colds and fevers to more complex conditions such as malaria and diabetes. Ground into powders, brewed into teas, or chewed raw, bitter kola offers a natural remedy for an assortment of health complaints, drawing upon the accumulated wisdom of generations past.

Folklore And Mythology Surrounding Bitter Kola

Entwined with the fabric of myth and folklore, bitter kola occupies a prominent place in the collective imagination of African cultures. Legends abound of ancient deities bestowing the gift of bitter kola upon humanity, imbuing it with mystical powers and divine blessings. According to folklore, the consumption of bitter kola confers protection from malevolent spirits, wards off misfortune, and ensures prosperity and longevity.

In many traditional societies, bitter kola is regarded as a sacred symbol of ancestral wisdom and spiritual enlightenment. Rituals and ceremonies centered around bitter kola are conducted to invoke the blessings of ancestral spirits, seek guidance in times of trouble, and celebrate the interconnectedness of life. Whether as a token of gratitude or an offering of reverence, bitter kola serves as a bridge between the material and spiritual realms, uniting past, present, and future in a timeless continuum of existence.

CHAPTER 2: BOTANICAL DESCRIPTION AND CLASSIFICATION

Taxonomy And Botanical Classification

Bitter kola, scientifically known as Garcinia kola, belongs to the family Clusiaceae, a diverse group of flowering plants commonly known as the mangosteen family. Within this family, Garcinia is a genus comprising over 200 species, many of which are indigenous to tropical regions of Asia, Africa, and Polynesia. The genus Garcinia is characterized by its evergreen trees and shrubs, glossy leaves, and fleshy fruits, which range in size, shape, and color across different species.

Botanical Description

Morphology: Bitter kola is a medium-sized evergreen tree that typically grows to a height of 10 to 20 meters (33 to 66 feet). Its trunk is straight, with smooth gray bark that may become slightly fissured with age. The tree branches profusely, forming a dense canopy of foliage consisting of elliptical leaves arranged in opposite pairs along the stems. The leaves are dark green and glossy, with prominent veins and entire margins. Each leaf measures about 5 to 10 centimeters (2 to 4 inches) in length and tapers to a pointed tip.

Flowers:

Bitter kola produces small, greenish-yellow flowers that are borne singly or in clusters in the leaf axils. The flowers are typically unisexual, with separate male and female individuals on the

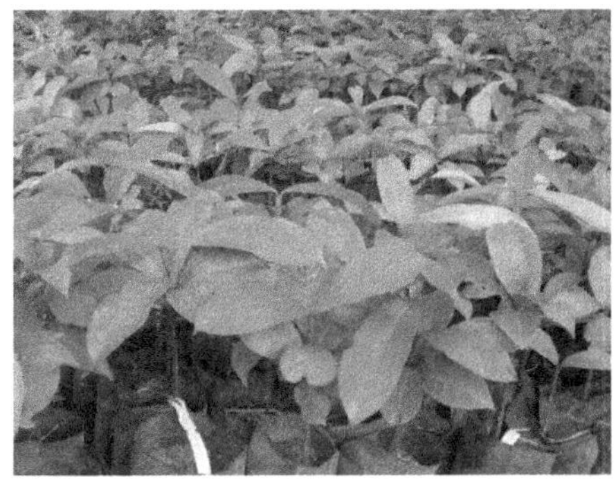

same tree (monoecious), although some trees may have bisexual flowers. The flowers are inconspicuous and lack petals, consisting of five sepals and numerous stamens or pistils. They are pollinated primarily by bees and other insects attracted to their nectar.

Fruits:

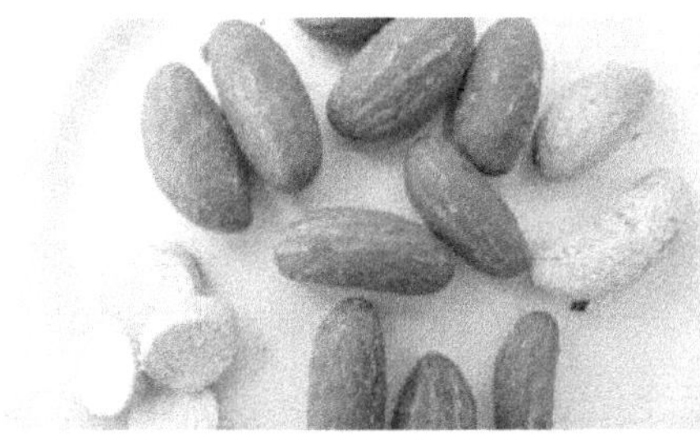

The fruit of bitter kola is a large, orange-colored berry with a hard, woody shell. It is roughly spherical in shape, measuring 5 to 10 centimeters (2 to 4 inches) in diameter, and contains several seeds embedded in a fibrous pulp. When ripe, the fruit splits open to reveal the seeds, which are enclosed in white, fleshy arils. These seeds are the source of bitter kola's medicinal properties and are traditionally used in various forms for therapeutic purposes.

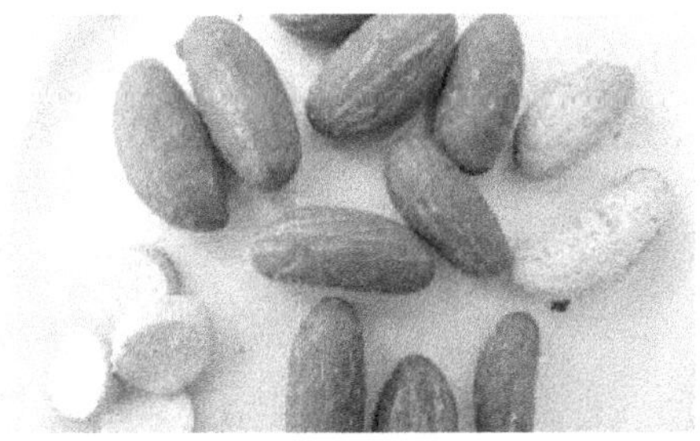

Reproductive Biology

Bitter kola is a perennial, woody plant with a long reproductive life cycle. Flowering typically occurs during the rainy season, when environmental conditions are favorable for pollination and fruit development. The flowers are pollinated primarily by bees and other insects, which visit the blossoms in search of nectar and inadvertently transfer pollen between flowers. After pollination, the ovaries develop into fruits, which mature over several months before ripening and dispersing their seeds.

Ecological Significance

Bitter kola plays a vital role in the ecology of tropical rainforests, where it serves as a food source for numerous wildlife species. The fruits are eagerly consumed by various mammals, birds, and insects, which play a crucial role in seed dispersal and germination. By dispersing the seeds to new locations, these animals help to maintain the genetic diversity of bitter kola populations and facilitate the regeneration of forest ecosystems.

In addition to its ecological significance, bitter kola contributes to the cultural heritage and traditional knowledge of indigenous communities. Its presence in the forest understory provides valuable resources for local populations, who have long relied on its medicinal properties for health and well-being. As stewards of the land, these communities play a vital role in conserving bitter kola and other medicinal plants, ensuring their continued availability for future generations.

CHAPTER 3: CHEMICAL COMPOSITION AND PHARMACOLOGICAL PROPERTIES OF BITTER KOLA

Phytochemicals And Active Compounds

Bitter kola is renowned for its rich array of phytochemicals, which contribute to its distinctive taste and potent medicinal properties. Among the most notable active compounds found in bitter kola are:

1. Alkaloids: Alkaloids are nitrogen-containing compounds with diverse physiological effects. Bitter kola contains several alkaloids, including kolaviron, kolanin, and garcinia biflavonoids. These alkaloids exhibit a wide range of pharmacological activities, including antioxidant, anti-inflammatory, and antimicrobial effects. Kolaviron, in particular, has been extensively studied for its potential therapeutic benefits in the treatment of various diseases.

2. Flavonoids: Flavonoids are a class of polyphenolic compounds with antioxidant and anti-inflammatory properties. Bitter kola contains flavonoids such as quercetin, kaempferol, and catechin, which contribute to its bitter taste and medicinal properties. These flavonoids have been shown to possess antioxidant activity, scavenging free radicals and protecting cells from oxidative damage. They may also help reduce inflammation and support cardiovascular health.

3. Tannins: Tannins are polyphenolic compounds that contribute to the astringent taste of bitter kola. They have been found to possess antimicrobial and anti-inflammatory properties, making them valuable for the treatment of various infections and inflammatory conditions. Tannins in bitter kola may help inhibit the growth of bacteria, fungi, and other pathogens, making it a useful natural remedy for gastrointestinal disorders and skin infections.

Analytical Techniques For Compound Identification

The chemical composition of bitter kola can be analyzed using a variety of analytical techniques, each offering unique insights into its phytochemical profile. Some of the most commonly used techniques include:

1. **High-Performance Liquid Chromatography (HPLC):** HPLC is a powerful analytical technique used to separate, identify, and quantify individual compounds in complex mixtures. By employing specialized columns and detectors, HPLC allows researchers to isolate specific phytochemicals in bitter kola extracts and measure their concentrations with high precision.

2. **Gas Chromatography-Mass Spectrometry (GC-MS):** GC-MS is another valuable technique for analyzing the chemical composition of bitter kola. It involves the separation of volatile compounds by gas chromatography, followed by their identification based on their mass spectra. GC-MS is particularly useful for detecting and quantifying volatile organic compounds and essential oils in bitter kola extracts.

3. **Nuclear Magnetic Resonance (NMR) Spectroscopy:** NMR spectroscopy is a non-destructive technique used to determine the structure and conformation of organic molecules. By subjecting bitter kola extracts to NMR analysis, researchers can elucidate the chemical structure of individual compounds and identify functional groups within complex mixtures.

Pharmacological Properties And Therapeutic Potential

Bitter kola possesses a wide range of pharmacological properties that contribute to its traditional use as a medicinal plant. Some of the most notable therapeutic effects of bitter kola include:

1. Antioxidant Activity: Bitter kola is rich in antioxidants, which help protect cells from oxidative damage caused by free radicals. These antioxidants may help reduce the risk of chronic diseases such as cancer, heart disease, and neurodegenerative disorders.

2. Anti-inflammatory Effects: Compounds found in bitter kola have been shown to possess anti-inflammatory properties, which may help reduce inflammation and alleviate symptoms of inflammatory conditions such as arthritis, asthma, and inflammatory bowel disease.

3. Antimicrobial and Antiparasitic Properties: Bitter kola contains compounds with antimicrobial and antiparasitic properties, which may help inhibit the growth of bacteria, fungi, and parasites. These properties make bitter kola a potential treatment for infections caused by pathogens such as bacteria, viruses, and protozoa.

4. Hepatoprotective Effects: Some studies suggest that bitter kola may have hepatoprotective effects, meaning it can help protect the liver from damage caused by toxins, drugs, or alcohol. This hepatoprotective activity may be attributed to the presence of bioactive compounds such as kolaviron, which has been shown to exhibit liver-protective properties in animal studies.

5. Anti-diabetic Effects: Bitter kola has been investigated for its potential anti-diabetic effects, with some studies suggesting that it may help regulate blood sugar levels and improve insulin sensitivity. These effects could be attributed to the presence of bioactive compounds such as kolaviron and garcinia biflavonoids, which have been shown to modulate glucose metabolism and insulin signaling pathways.

CHAPTER 4: TRADITIONAL USES IN AFRICAN MEDICINE

Historical Context Of Medicinal Plant Use

The utilization of bitter kola within traditional African medicine is deeply rooted in the continent's cultural heritage and indigenous knowledge systems. Across diverse ethnic groups and regions, the practice of herbalism has been integral to healthcare for generations. Traditional healers, often revered as custodians of ancient wisdom, have passed down knowledge of medicinal plants, including bitter kola, through oral traditions and practical apprenticeships.

Traditional Remedies and Healing Practices

The traditional uses of bitter kola are as diverse as the cultures that embrace it. From Nigeria to Cameroon, Ghana to the Democratic Republic of the Congo, bitter kola has been employed in a multitude of remedies to address a wide spectrum of health concerns. These include:

- **Respiratory Conditions:** Bitter kola is traditionally used to alleviate symptoms of respiratory infections such as coughs, colds, and bronchitis. Its expectorant properties help loosen phlegm and clear airways, while its antimicrobial effects may assist in combating the underlying infection.

- **Digestive Disorders:** Bitter kola is valued for its ability to aid digestion and soothe gastrointestinal discomfort. It is employed to treat conditions ranging from indigestion and flatulence to dysentery and diarrhea. The bitter taste of the seeds is believed to stimulate digestive juices and promote proper digestion.

- **Sexual Health:** Bitter kola is reputed for its aphrodisiac properties and is used to enhance sexual function and libido. It is believed to increase arousal, improve erectile function, and enhance fertility in both men and women. These effects are attributed to compounds in bitter kola that may influence hormonal balance and blood flow.

- **Malaria Management:** Bitter kola is a staple in the traditional treatment of malaria and febrile illnesses. Its antipyretic properties help reduce fever, while its antimalarial effects may aid in combating the parasite responsible for the disease. Bitter kola is often included in herbal remedies alongside other plants with anti-malarial properties.

Bitter Kola In Rituals And Ceremonies

Beyond its medicinal uses, bitter kola holds profound cultural and spiritual significance in African societies. It is frequently incorporated into rituals and ceremonies to invoke blessings, protection, and communal harmony. Bitter kola is used as an offering in ceremonies such as weddings, births, and funerals, symbolizing prosperity, fertility, and ancestral reverence. Its bitter taste is believed to cleanse and purify, while its presence is thought to attract benevolent spirits and ensure the success of communal endeavors.

14

CHAPTER 5: PHARMACOLOGICAL PROPERTIES AND THERAPEUTIC POTENTIAL

Antioxidant Activity And Free Radical Scavenging

Bitter kola's antioxidant properties are attributed to its rich content of bioactive compounds, including flavonoids, tannins, and phenolic acids. These compounds neutralize free radicals, reactive molecules that can damage cells and contribute to aging and disease. By scavenging free radicals, bitter kola helps protect cells from oxidative stress and reduces the risk of chronic diseases such as cancer, cardiovascular disease, and neurodegenerative disorders.

Anti-Inflammatory And Analgesic Effects

Compounds in bitter kola possess anti-inflammatory properties, which can help reduce inflammation and alleviate pain. Inflammation is a natural immune response that can become chronic and contribute to various diseases, including arthritis, asthma, and inflammatory bowel disease. Bitter kola's anti-inflammatory effects are mediated by its ability to inhibit pro-inflammatory enzymes and cytokines, thereby modulating the inflammatory response and promoting tissue healing.

Antimicrobial And Antiparasitic Properties

Bitter kola exhibits broad-spectrum antimicrobial activity against bacteria, fungi, viruses, and parasites. Its antimicrobial properties are attributed to compounds such as kolaviron, kolanin, and garcinia biflavonoids, which disrupt microbial cell membranes, inhibit enzyme activity, and interfere with nucleic acid synthesis. Bitter kola's antiparasitic effects are particularly noteworthy in the context of malaria, as it has been shown to inhibit the growth of Plasmodium spp., the parasites responsible for the disease.

Cardioprotective Effects

Bitter kola has potential cardioprotective effects, which may help prevent and manage cardiovascular diseases such as hypertension, atherosclerosis, and heart failure. Its cardiovascular benefits are attributed to its ability to lower blood pressure, reduce cholesterol levels, and improve blood vessel function. Bitter kola also possesses antiplatelet and antithrombotic properties, which can help prevent blood clots and reduce the risk of heart attack and stroke.

Neuroprotective Effects

Compounds in bitter kola exhibit neuroprotective properties, which may help prevent and mitigate neurodegenerative diseases such as Alzheimer's and Parkinson's disease. Bitter kola's neuroprotective effects are attributed to its ability to inhibit the formation of amyloid-beta plaques and tau protein tangles, which are hallmarks of Alzheimer's disease. Additionally, bitter kola protects neurons from oxidative stress and inflammation, thereby preserving cognitive function and promoting brain health.

Immunomodulatory Effects

Bitter kola modulates the immune system, enhancing its ability to defend against infections and diseases. It stimulates the production of immune cells such as macrophages, lymphocytes, and natural killer cells, which play a crucial role in identifying and eliminating pathogens. Bitter kola also enhances the production of cytokines and antibodies, which regulate immune responses and promote immune function.

CHAPTER 6: SIDE EFFECTS AND CONTRAINDICATIONS

Bitter Kola And Potential Side Effects

While bitter kola is generally considered safe when consumed in moderation, prolonged or excessive use may lead to certain side effects. These side effects can vary depending on individual factors such as dosage, duration of use, and overall health status:

- **Digestive Disturbances:** Excessive consumption of bitter kola may lead to gastrointestinal discomfort, including symptoms such as nausea, vomiting, abdominal pain, and bloating. These effects are primarily attributed to the presence of tannins, which can irritate the digestive tract and disrupt normal gut function.

- **Allergic Reactions:** Some individuals may experience allergic reactions to bitter kola, particularly if they have sensitivities to its active compounds. Allergic symptoms may include skin rashes, itching, swelling of the face or throat, difficulty breathing, or anaphylaxis in severe cases. Individuals with known allergies to plants in the Clusiaceae family should exercise caution when using bitter kola.

- **Interactions with Medications:** Bitter kola may interact with certain medications, potentially affecting their efficacy or increasing the risk of adverse effects. For example, bitter kola has been reported to interact with anticoagulant drugs such as warfarin, leading to an increased risk of bleeding. It may also interact with medications for diabetes, hypertension, and psychiatric disorders. Individuals taking prescription medications should consult with a healthcare professional before using bitter kola.

- **Pregnancy and Breastfeeding:** The safety of bitter kola during pregnancy and breastfeeding is not well established. While traditional use suggests potential benefits for maternal and fetal health, there is limited scientific evidence to support its safety in these populations. Pregnant and breastfeeding women should exercise caution and consult with a healthcare provider before using bitter kola.

Contraindications And Precautions

Certain populations may be advised to avoid or use caution when using bitter kola due to underlying health conditions or potential risks:

- **Gastrointestinal Disorders:** Individuals with pre existing gastrointestinal conditions such as ulcers, gastritis, or irritable bowel syndrome (IBS) may experience worsening symptoms with bitter kola consumption. The high tannin content of bitter kola seeds can exacerbate gastric irritation and lead to gastrointestinal distress. Individuals with these conditions should consult with a healthcare professional before using bitter kola.

- **Bleeding Disorders:** Bitter kola contains compounds that may affect blood clotting and platelet function, potentially increasing the risk of bleeding in individuals with bleeding disorders such as hemophilia or thrombocytopenia. These individuals should use caution when consuming bitter kola and discuss potential risks with a healthcare provider.

- **Liver and Kidney Conditions:** Bitter kola may have hepatoprotective effects in some cases, but individuals with liver or kidney conditions should use caution and consult with a healthcare provider before using bitter kola. The interaction between bitter kola and medications used to treat liver or kidney disease is not well understood, and there may be potential risks associated with its use in these populations.

- **Allergies:** Individuals with known allergies to plants in the Clusiaceae family, such as mangosteen or garcinia, may be at increased risk of allergic reactions to bitter kola. These individuals should avoid bitter kola and seek alternative remedies to avoid potential adverse effects.

CHAPTER 7: FUTURE DIRECTIONS FOR RESEARCH

Exploring Novel Therapeutic Applications

As scientific interest in natural remedies grows, there is increasing exploration of the potential therapeutic applications of bitter kola beyond its traditional uses. Future research may focus on:

- **Cancer Prevention and Treatment:** Preliminary studies suggest that bitter kola may possess anti-cancer properties, including inhibition of tumor growth and induction of cancer cell death. Future research may investigate the mechanisms of action underlying these effects and evaluate the potential of bitter kola as an adjunctive therapy for cancer prevention and treatment.

- **Metabolic Disorders:** Bitter kola has shown promise in modulating glucose metabolism and insulin sensitivity, suggesting potential benefits for individuals with diabetes and metabolic syndrome. Future studies may explore the effects of bitter kola on blood sugar regulation, lipid metabolism, and obesity-related complications, as well as its potential role in preventing and managing metabolic disorders.

- **Neurological Disorders:** Bitter kola's neuroprotective effects have implications for the prevention and management of neurodegenerative diseases such as Alzheimer's and Parkinson's disease. Research may focus on elucidating the mechanisms by which bitter kola protects neurons from oxidative stress and inflammation, as well as its potential for cognitive enhancement and neuroregeneration.

- **Antimicrobial Resistance:** Bitter kola's antimicrobial properties make it a promising candidate for combating antimicrobial resistance, a global health threat. Future studies may investigate its efficacy against drug-resistant pathogens and explore novel therapeutic strategies, such as combination therapies and synergistic effects with conventional antibiotics.

Standardization And Quality Control

To ensure the safety, efficacy, and reproducibility of bitter kola-based therapies, there is a need for standardization and quality control measures in production and manufacturing. Future research may involve:

- **Development of Standardized Extracts:** Standardized extracts of bitter kola can help ensure consistent dosing and potency across different formulations. Research may focus on optimizing extraction methods, identifying bioactive compounds, and establishing quality control parameters for commercial products.

- **Quality Assurance and Authentication:** Methods for verifying the authenticity and purity of bitter kola products are essential for safeguarding consumer health and preventing adulteration or contamination. Research may explore techniques such as DNA barcoding, chromatographic fingerprinting, and spectroscopic analysis for quality assurance and authentication.

- **Regulatory Frameworks and Guidelines:** Establishing regulatory frameworks and guidelines for the production, labeling, and marketing of bitter kola products can help ensure compliance with safety and quality standards. Collaboration between regulatory agencies, industry stakeholders, and scientific experts is needed to develop evidence-based guidelines and best practices.

Community Engagement And Knowledge Translation

Engaging with local communities and traditional healers is crucial for promoting the sustainable use of bitter kola and preserving indigenous knowledge. Future research may involve:

- **Community-Based Participatory Research:** Collaborative research partnerships with local communities can help ensure that research priorities align with community needs and values. Engaging community members as active participants in research design, implementation, and dissemination can enhance the relevance and impact of research outcomes.

- **Knowledge Translation and Capacity Building:** Efforts to translate scientific findings into accessible formats and disseminate them to relevant stakeholders can help bridge the gap between research and practice. Capacity-building initiatives, such as training programs and educational materials, can empower traditional healers and healthcare providers to integrate evidence-based practices into their work and promote informed decision-making among consumers.

CHAPTER 8: SOCIETAL, CULTURAL, AND ECONOMIC IMPLICATIONS

Bitter Kola In Socio-Cultural Context

The significance of bitter kola extends beyond its medicinal properties to encompass broader socio-cultural dimensions. In many African societies, bitter kola plays a central role in social interactions, rituals, and ceremonies. It is often exchanged as a customary gift during weddings, births, and other auspicious occasions, symbolizing hospitality, goodwill, and mutual respect. Bitter kola is also deeply ingrained in spiritual practices, where it is believed to possess protective and purifying qualities. Its bitter taste is metaphorically associated with life's challenges and the resilience required to overcome them, making it a potent symbol of strength and endurance.

Economic Opportunities And Challenges

The cultivation and trade of bitter kola represent important economic activities in many regions of Africa, providing livelihoods for thousands of people along the supply chain. Smallholder farmers rely on bitter kola cultivation as a source of income, while traders, processors, and retailers contribute to the value chain through marketing and distribution. However, the bitter kola industry faces several challenges, including fluctuating market prices, limited access to markets, and lack of infrastructure for processing and storage. Additionally, unsustainable harvesting practices and deforestation pose threats to the long-term viability of bitter kola production, highlighting the need for sustainable management practices and conservation efforts.

Health Equity And Access

Despite its widespread use in traditional medicine, bitter kola's potential health benefits remain underutilized and often inaccessible to marginalized communities. Socioeconomic disparities, inadequate healthcare infrastructure, and limited access to information contribute to disparities in health outcomes and access to healthcare services. Addressing these barriers requires a multi-faceted approach that prioritizes health equity, community engagement, and capacity-building initiatives. By promoting the integration of traditional medicine into primary healthcare systems and supporting community-led health initiatives, bitter kola can play a pivotal role in advancing health equity and improving health outcomes for underserved populations.

CHAPTER 8: CONCLUSION

In conclusion, bitter kola stands as a testament to the rich tapestry of Africa's botanical heritage, embodying centuries of traditional knowledge, cultural significance, and medicinal wisdom. Its bitter taste and potent medicinal properties have earned it a revered place in indigenous healing traditions, where it continues to play a vital role in promoting health and well-being.

As we look towards the future, it is imperative that we embrace a holistic approach to the study and utilization of bitter kola, one that recognizes its ecological, socio-cultural, and economic dimensions. Sustainable management practices, conservation efforts, and community-driven initiatives are essential for safeguarding bitter kola's biodiversity and ensuring its availability for future generations.

Furthermore, continued research into the pharmacological properties, therapeutic applications, and safety profile of bitter kola is crucial for unlocking its full potential as a natural remedy. By investing in scientific inquiry, innovation, and knowledge-sharing, we can harness the healing power of bitter kola to address pressing health challenges and improve the well-being of individuals and communities worldwide.

In this journey towards a sustainable future, collaboration and partnership are key. By fostering dialogue, building bridges between traditional knowledge and modern science, and fostering inclusive approaches to healthcare, we can cultivate a more equitable and resilient healthcare system that honors the wisdom of the past while embracing the opportunities of the future.

As we embark on this collective endeavor, let us remain mindful of the ethical responsibilities and stewardship duties that accompany our exploration of bitter kola and other medicinal plants. Let us tread lightly on the earth, respecting the delicate balance of ecosystems, and honoring the cultural heritage and sacred traditions that bind us to the natural world.

In the spirit of ubuntu, let us strive to be good stewards of bitter kola and all living beings, recognizing that our collective well-being is intricately interconnected with the health of the planet. Together, let us embark on a journey of discovery, healing, and renewal, guided by the wisdom of bitter kola and the enduring spirit of resilience that defines us as a people.

GLOSSARY

1. **Phytochemicals:** Chemical compounds produced by plants, often possessing biological activity and health benefits. Examples include flavonoids, alkaloids, and tannins.

2. **Antioxidants:** Molecules that inhibit the oxidation of other molecules, thus protecting cells from damage caused by free radicals.

3. **Aphrodisiac:** Substances believed to increase sexual desire or libido.

4. **Antipyretic:** Medications or substances that reduce fever.

5. **Hepatoprotective:** Agents that protect the liver from damage and promote its healing.

6. **Neuroprotective:** Substances that protect neurons from damage or degeneration.

7. **Antimicrobial:** Agents that kill or inhibit the growth of microorganisms such as bacteria, viruses, fungi, or parasites.

8. **Antiparasitic:** Agents that kill or inhibit the growth of parasites.

9. **Anti-inflammatory:** Substances that reduce inflammation, swelling, and pain.

10. **Hypertension:** High blood pressure, a condition associated with increased risk of heart disease and stroke.

REFERENCES

1. Atawodi SE. (2009). Nigerian foodstuffs with prostate cancer chemopreventive polyphenols. *Discov Innov.*

2. Farombi EO, Adepoju BF, Ola-Davies OE, Emerole GO, Nwankwo JO. (2016). *Bitter kola (Garcinia kola) inhibits pancreatic cancer cell growth and induces apoptosis: Involvement of mitochondrial pathways.*

3. Gbadamosi IT, Salawu SO, Lasisi AA, et al. (2012). Anti-inflammatory and analgesic effects of aqueous extract of Garcinia kola seed in experimental animals. *African Journal of Traditional, Complementary, and Alternative Medicines.*

4. Ghosh R, Nadiminty N, Fitzpatrick JE, Alworth WL, Slaga TJ, Kumar AP. (2010). Eugenol causes melanoma growth suppression through inhibition of E2F1 transcriptional activity. *Journal of Biological Chemistry.*

5. Okunji CO, Iwu MM. (2003). Medicinal plants of Nigeria: a preliminary survey of plants used in Nigerian ethnomedicine. *Journal of Ethnopharmacology.*

6. Olajide OA, Awe SO, Makinde JM, Ekhelar AI, Olusola A, Morebise O. (1999). Evaluation of the anti-inflammatory properties of the hexane extract of Garcinia kola seed. *Journal of Ethnopharmacology.*

7. Osuagwu FC, Oladele AA, Akinola OB, Oremosu AA, Olajide OA. (2011). Garcinia kola seeds aqueous extract and its fractions attenuate inflammatory cytokines-induced pain in rodents. *Journal of Ethnopharmacology.*

8. Sani Y, Muhammad AU, Yaro AH, Musa KY. (2013). Antibacterial activity of Garcinia kola seeds on some

food-borne pathogens. *American Journal of Research Communication.*

9. Sofowora A. (1993). Medicinal Plants and Traditional Medicine in Africa. *Chichester: John Wiley & Sons.*

10. Tona L, Ngimbi NP, Tsakala M, Mesia K, Cimanga K, Apers S, et al. (1999). Antimalarial activity of 20 crude extracts from nine African medicinal plants used in Kinshasa, Congo. *Journal of Ethnopharmacology.*

ABOUT THE AUTHOR

Egbo Daniel

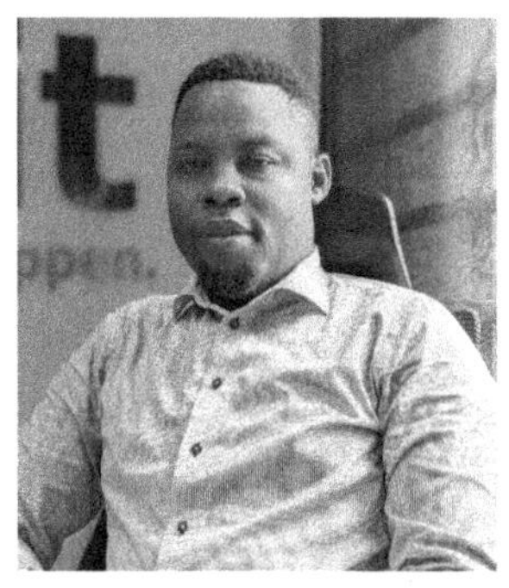

Egbo Daniel, a prodigious young researcher, a fervent follower and student of Dr. Sebi (Alfredo Darrington Bowman), the great Herbal Guru and fervent advocate for natural remedies, stands at the forefront of exploring the intersection between traditional knowledge and modern science. With an insatiable curiosity and a deep-rooted belief in the healing power of nature, Egbo Daniel has dedicated their budding career to unravelling the mysteries of botanical medicine.

Egbo Daniel has already made significant strides in the field, earning recognition for groundbreaking research that bridges the gap between ancient wisdom and contemporary healthcare practices. His passion for uncovering the therapeutic potential of natural compounds has propelled him to the forefront of a new generation of scientists committed to holistic approaches to wellness.

With a commitment to sustainability and a reverence for indigenous knowledge, Egbo Daniel strives to promote the integration of natural remedies into mainstream healthcare, offering a holistic perspective that honours both tradition and innovation. Through this work, he seeks to inspire others to explore the rich tapestry of nature's offerings and harness its healing power for the betterment of humanity.

Egbo Daniel holds a deep-seated belief in the transformative potential of natural remedies, viewing them not only as alternatives to conventional pharmaceuticals but as integral components of a balanced and harmonious approach to health and well-being. As he continue to chart new territory in the realm of botanical medicine, Egbo Daniel remains steadfast in their dedication to advancing the field and empowering individuals to take control of their health through the wonders of nature's pharmacy.

BOOKS IN THIS SERIES

HEALTH SERIES

A SERIES OF WORKS ON HEALTHY LIVING AND CARE FOR THE BODY ESPECIALLY AS RELATES TO NATURAL REMEDIES AGAINST DRUGS, SUPPLEMENTS AND OTHER SCIENTIFIC PRODUCTS

The Medicinal Properties Of Bitter Kola And Its Potential Health Benefits